GROWING UP & GLOWING UP

A Girl's Guide to Well Being

By Dr. Mary Ann Yehl

THIS BOOK IS DEDICATED
TO MY LOVING FAMILY.

Contents

CHAPTER 1

~ ❖ ~

What Happens Inside a Girl's Body?

"YOU MUST ALWAYS HAVE
FAITH IN PEOPLE. AND MOST
IMPORTANTLY, YOU MUST ALWAYS
HAVE FAITH IN YOURSELF."
-ELLE WOODS, LEGALLY
BLONDE

*O*nce women enter pre-teen ages, their bodies start to change in ways that can be exciting, confusing, and scary, especially if you are unprepared.

This book was made to help you understand why the changes happen, what they will look like, and the fact that there are many differences in our bodies that are completely normal. Not all women look the same, and that is a good thing.

We want to embrace our differences and respect our bodies for what they allow us to do– think, see, hear, move, exercise, laugh!

Let's take a look at what happens every month and the reasons why it happens.

The Anatomy of Females

- Breast
- Uterus/Fallopian Tubes/Ovaries
- Vagina (inside)
- Vulva or Labia (outside)

Puberty is the beginning of changes; for girls, it starts between 8–12 years old and takes years.

Normal things that happen during puberty – pimples, hair in armpits, some body odor develops, hair in private parts.

1.1. Breast development

- It can take years for breasts to fully develop and can be a little sensitive or uncomfortable during this time.
- It is normal for most women to have one bigger breast, sometimes a lot bigger– please go to your healthcare provider if you have concerns or questions.
- Breasts are made up of breast tissue (the soft, squishy part), nipple (the part that sticks out sometimes– tip), and areola (the circular darker part surrounding the nipple).

- Nipples can vary greatly in shape and size and that's normal – some women have larger nipples like the tip of a finger, and others have smaller nipples like the tip of a pencil.

- Areolas also vary greatly in size and color, some are very light and some very dark in color, and some are the size of a quarter and some are the size of a coffee mug.

> **Pro tip** – don't buy expensive bras because breast size can change throughout puberty and also with weight gain/loss.

1.2. Lower half anatomy

- You are born with the parts – nothing new is generated during puberty, only new functions arise.

- Outside parts of the vagina – vulva are the folds of skin on the outside, they may get bigger or get a darker color during puberty.

- Vulva also looks different in all women, some have more skin, or thicker skin, down there, and some have looser skin or darker coloring.
    - There are three outlets down there for girls – starting from the front to back with what comes out of each opening;
        - Urethral opening – urine
        - Vagina – mucous, period blood, and babies
        - Rectum – poop
    - They are not connected in any way, just next door to one another.

Girl's bodies have an order of development:

Once you get a period, it can be pretty erratic and irregular for the first year or so.

Your body tells the brain what hormones must be released to make certain functions happen for specific reasons.

The menstrual cycle has two parts, the follicular and the luteal; and a lot of actions that happen in these parts begin around hormones.

What are hormones?

Great communicators. They are chemical messengers that send signals through the blood into muscles and tissues of the body.

The following are the actions of hormones:

- They signal when and how things in the body should happen.
- Hormones are given directions by organs and endocrine glands.

There are over 50 hormones in the body.

Examples of hormones include insulin, estrogen, testosterone, cortisol, etc.

Their wide array of jobs includes growth and development, metabolism, controlling mood, sexual functioning, sleep cycle, reproduction, etc.

The hormones we will talk about related to girls are:

Hormone	Job
Estrogen	signals many areas of the body for pregnancy, helps maintain regular periods, and improves bone health
Progesterone	gets the uterus ready for pregnancy and the breast ready for milk production. Also, a quick drop in this hormone every month causes period bleeding
Follicle Stimulating Hormone	gets the follicle (egg) in the ovary ready to release into the uterus
Luteinizing Hormone	controls the production of estrogen from ovaries, signals when to release the follicle (egg) into the uterus

Below is a picture of one side of the female internal reproductive organs:

- The uterus in the middle – this is where the lining builds up and sheds every month, and it is where a baby grows if there is a pregnancy.

- The cervix in the bottom part of the uterus – this is the area that is used for Pap smear testing.

- The ovary – this is where the eggs are stored and where the follicle develops and is released every month.

- The Fallopian tube – this is where the follicle travels through to the uterus.

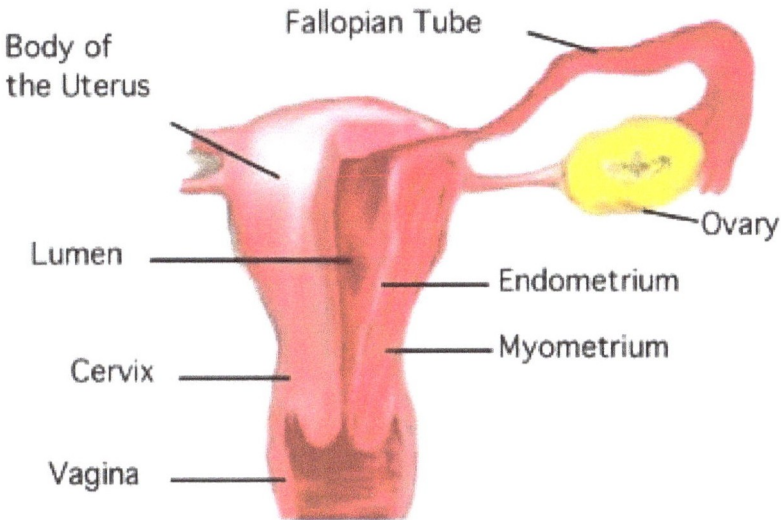

Body of the Uterus

Fallopian Tube

Ovary

Lumen

Endometrium

Myometrium

Cervix

Vagina

Teixiera et al ,2008

The Menstrual Cycle Chart

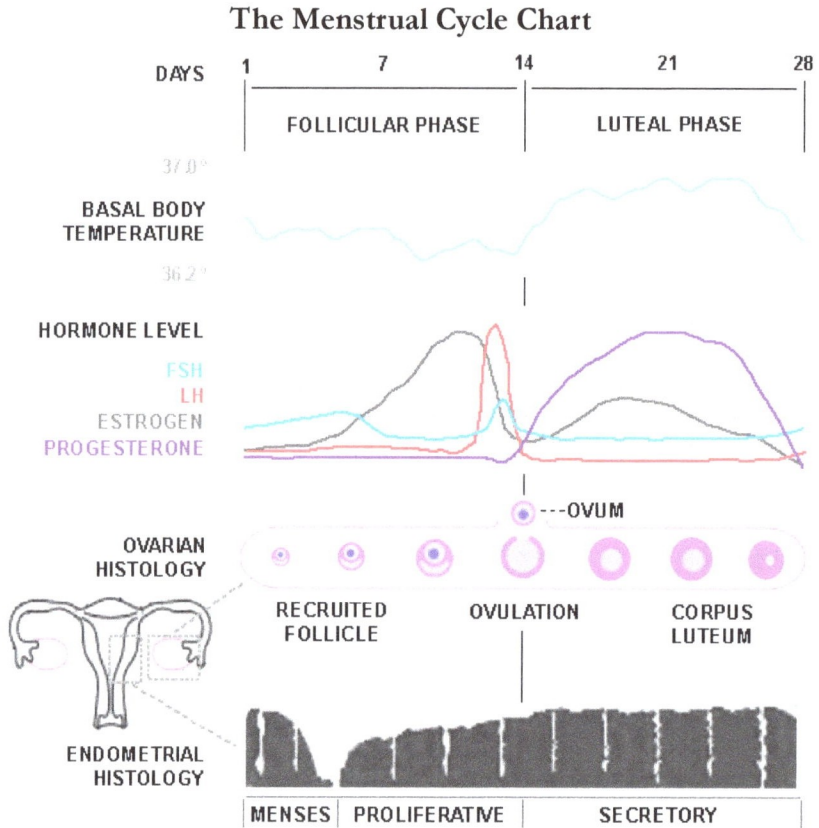

Isometrik, 2008

The Follicular Phase

- This phase starts with Day 1 of your period and ends with ovulation (around day 14).

- Three hormones come into play in this phase of the cycle – estrogen, FSH, and LH.

- First, the body releases estrogen with levels slowly rising, which helps thicken the inside or lining of the uterus. The idea behind this is the uterus is getting ready in case there is a pregnancy.

- Next, FSH is released which signals a follicle (egg) to get ready to be released from the ovary and the LH signals the moment of release and the subsequent travel towards the uterus through the connecting tube (Fallopian tube). This is around day 14 for the average woman.

The Luteal Phase

- This is between days 15 to 28.

- The estrogen levels decrease and the progesterone levels increase.

- Now, the egg travels from the tube into the uterus, as progesterone helps the uterus lining prepare in case of implantation (if the egg meets a sperm and is fertilized, resulting in pregnancy).

- If that does not happen, the level of progesterone drops, and a period starts.

Vaginal Discharge

- Vaginal discharge is a normal part of the female cycle.

- It changes throughout the cycle in amount and consistency.

- Why? The cells in the vagina secrete fluid for two reasons – to clean out old cells and debris and to lubricate the vagina.

  - Days 1–7 (period days); minimal discharge, bleeding from red to dark red to brownish color.

  - Days 7–14; discharge starts as clear or white, thin, and watery then during ovulation changes to an egg-white consistency, usually a larger amount of discharge, noticeable most days.

  - Day 14–28; thin, clear-to-white discharge, more watery in consistency.

- See a healthcare provider if your vaginal discharge:

  - Smells really bad or fishy

  - Color has changed – from normal to bright yellow, green, gray, etc.

  - Consistency has changed – from normal to cottage cheese.

  - Amount has changed – from normal to suddenly soaking underwear.

- Is combined with bleeding, itching, burning, or rashes

Breast Changes

- During different times of your cycle, it is normal to have some mild breast discomfort or tenderness.
- What is not normal – intense pain, lumps, discharge, or redness – See your healthcare provider right away.

Pro tip – getting your period every month should not stop your life in any way It is time to get checked if you have :

- Severe menstrual cramps/pain.
- Intense mood changes.

Questions

Do you know when you are ovulating?

Some women have a little cramp on the lower belly, right or left side, bloating, or a spot of blood, but it is very unpredictable.

Can you prevent ovulation?

Yes with hormones – taking pills, shots, or using hormones inside the uterus.

What is a normal period?

It occurs every 21–35 days and can vary each month.

The bleeding with a period can last anywhere from 2–7 days.

The amount is about 2–3 tablespoons or 80 mL.

What is a tampon?

A tampon is a piece of cotton (usually) with a piece of attached thick string that is inserted through the vagina – its job is to stay inside the vagina and absorb the blood from a period for 4–6 hours.

You remove the tampon by pulling on the string.

You then put it in the garbage or the sanitary containers in the bathroom (wrap it in toilet paper first).

DO NOT FLUSH TAMPONS, they clog drains like crazy.

When do you *need* to see a healthcare provider?

No period by age 15

You have a period and then it stops.

You have a lot of pain during your cycle.

The amount of bleeding is heavy (soaking one pad per hour for a few hours).

You *can* see a doctor or your healthcare provider anytime for any questions or concerns.

Is there anything I can do to help with cramping?

Over-the-counter medicines like ibuprofen can help with cramps.

Can I take medicine to stop a period?

Yes, prescribed hormones.

Do I have to stop doing any activities when I have a period?

No.

Can I swim, shower, and take a bath with my period?

Yes.

Can anyone tell if I have my period?

No.

Does a period smell bad?

No, it shouldn't. A period is made up of blood and tissues and smells like blood. You will start to notice the same smell every month with your period. If you experience a different smell than your normal period or a very strong or bad odor, please see your healthcare provider.

Do we need to get a period every month to be healthy?

Getting a period every month does tell you that your hormones and female systems are working well, so that is healthy.

If you are taking medicine by a healthcare provider that makes your periods super light or stop– is that ok?

YES, there is no reason you NEED a period to keep your body healthy every month – IF you are taking medicine that lessens or stops it.

If a period stops without you doing anything, please see your healthcare provider.

OK, so that was the bleeding part. Let's talk about the other things that happen to your body besides bleeding during the month.

Interactive Parts:

- What was the best compliment you have ever received?

- What is your favorite thing to do with friends?

- If you had to be an animal- which one would you be?

CHAPTER 2

~ ❖ ~

Deeper Dive into the Menstrual Cycle; Optimization

"NEVER DULL YOUR SHINE FOR SOMEBODY ELSE."
– **TYRA BANKS**

There is a lot of research about what happens in each cycle with hormones and energy. The research is a little grayer on exactly how diet and exercise affect the cycle patterns though. We know paying attention to YOUR body and YOUR symptoms, and eating and exercising so that YOU feel well works pretty well. Apps work really well for tracking both periods and symptoms that tag along with your cycle. Pay attention to energy, sleep, mood, hunger, cravings, headaches, cramps, etc., and when they occur.

Follicular Phase-Menstrual Days (Days 1–7)

- Symptoms are cramping, bleeding, being tired, moody, trouble sleeping, bloating, breast tenderness.

- Bleeding is happening – for most women, the bleeding isn't enough to cause low iron (iron is found in the blood). So for most women (without other medical issues), taking in a little extra iron-rich food is ok – foods like red meats, and green leafy veggies (think kale, and spinach).

- Magnesium is a great supplement for this phase (as it is for most phases) because it can help with headaches, bloating, and sleep.

- Foods – those that have magnesium are pumpkin seeds, peanuts almonds, spinach, black beans, and dark chocolate.

- Exercise – you may not feel like doing heavy exercises at this time, try yoga/stretching, long walks, and pilates instead.

Follicular Phase (Days 8–13)

- This phase starts with feelings of low energy but this later increases.

- Mood increases are there is the feeling of being more social/outgoing.

- Estrogen levels are high.

- Foods – balance high estrogen with cruciferous veggies (broccoli, cauliflower), flaxseed, green tea, berries, and healthy fats (avocado, salmon).

- Exercise – as energy levels increase, cardio can feel easier, and performance improves.

Ovulation Day (Day 14 ish)

- This is typically when we feel the best – confident, relaxed, energized, attractive.

- Don't forget this is when your body is ready to get pregnant (even if you don't want to) – so you feel confident, attractive, and social.

- Exercise – high energy makes performance very good – peaking around now.

Luteal Phase (Days 15–28)

- We see progesterone go up and then rapidly go down in this phase.

- Symptoms this causes are increased and then decreased energy, PMS (pre-menstrual syndrome).

- Symptoms towards the end of this phase – breast tenderness, bloating, cramping.

- Foods – if PMS symptoms arise and hunger and cravings are stronger – it is important to drink adequate water, and eat fiber-rich foods (veggies/fruits, whole grains (wheat breads, brown rice, quinoa), berries) to help avoid cravings and hunger.

- Serotonin (a chemical messenger that makes us feel happy) levels go down. Foods that help – chicken, eggs, fruits and veggies, and foods with omega 3 fatty acids like salmon, and nuts.

- Exercise – High energy exercises– HIT, spinning, racing, boot camp

Interactive Parts:

- Describe your perfect day?

- Do you prefer mountains or beaches?

- In 10 years, where do you see yourself living?

CHAPTER 3

~ ❖ ~

Period Problems

> "NOTE TO SELF:
> SELF-LOVE ISN'T SELFISH."
> **–DUA LIPA**

What can change the menstrual cycle or periods?

- Pregnancy

- Medical Conditions – hormonal issues (polycystic ovaries, fibroids, endometriosis), infections, ovary issues, eating disorders, excessive exercise, weight changes, drug use.

- There are many medical conditions that can affect your cycle, so it is important to get checked by a healthcare provider if your cycle isn't there or is very irregular.

What is abnormal with periods?

1. Period pain

- Normal periods can cause some mild cramps that last for a day or two.

- Abnormal (Dysmenorrhea) – Periods that have severe pain and sometimes also have nausea, headaches, vomiting, dizziness, severe fatigue, and mood changes.

- Treatment – go see your healthcare provider, there can be many reasons for this and you want to make sure you figure out why this happens to you.

- Home treatment – over-the-counter medicines like ibuprofen can help relieve symptoms (read the bottle for instructions on dosages), most women take these medicines for 1–2 days to feel better.

- Prescription medicines – your healthcare provider may give medicines with hormones, like birth control pills to alleviate these symptoms, as they stop ovulation so a regular period doesn't happen.

- Sometimes providers recommend taking birth control pills continuously and avoiding having any bleeding to help symptoms (some intrauterine devices or IUDs can also cause very infrequent bleeding or no bleeding – which is OK).

2. Abnormal Bleeding

- *Period missing (Amenorrhea)*
  - Most women have a period by the age of 12, but if you are 15 and have never had a period – go see your healthcare provider.

- *Period too irregularly (Oligomenorrhea)*
  - In your teen years, periods can be irregular, especially in that first year.
  - Normal periods come every 21–45 days and last 2–7 days.
  - Make sure that if you are having abnormal periods, you track it with an app and go see your healthcare provider.

- *Periods too long (Metrorrhagia)*
  - If a period lasts more than 7 days – that is too long.
  - Go to see your healthcare provider.

- *Period too heavy (Menorrhagia)*
  - Normal period blood amount using 3–6 pads or tampons per day (about 80 mL of blood).
  - If you find that a pad/tampon does not last 4 hours – it is completely soaked more than one time and you may leak through it – go see your healthcare provider.

3. Your period was here and now stopped

- Make sure you are accurately tracking this with an app.(See the resource list at the end)
- Irregular periods can be common in the first year after getting a period but if it has been regular and then you have skipped periods, by the 3rd time of skipped periods, go see your healthcare provider (of course if you are sexually active and suspect pregnancy – please test for that).

- Periods may stop in athletes who are training a lot and not eating enough– this is NOT ok; if this happens, go see your healthcare provider.

What is toxic shock syndrome?

- Toxic shock syndrome can be caused by leaving a tampon in too long and having a bacterial infection that goes throughout the body.

- It is a very severe infection that gives people fever, chills, pain, and rashes – if you think you may have left a tampon in or can't find a tampon you put in, please go see a healthcare provider right away.

- Tampons are meant to be used for 4–6 hours or so, don't use them overnight.

- If you are a person who has trouble remembering when you need to take a tampon out – don't use them or set an alarm on your phone to remind you.

- Tampons can't travel anywhere else inside the body once you put it in the vagina – they don't end up in the uterus or the abdomen.

Pro tip – if you are having trouble removing a tampon, or if you did forget to take it out for a few days – go see your healthcare provider right away.

Where to find care?

When do you need a pelvic exam or to see a gynecologist or have an exam "down there"?

- Anytime you are having concerns or issues (urinary issues, vaginal discharge, irregular periods, need birth control, need testing for sexually transmitted infections or (STIs)).

- Just because you see a doctor doesn't mean you will need a pelvic exam.

- It is a good idea to go BEFORE you become sexually active to have a plan and have your questions answered.

- You can talk about family history and figure out if you need any testing or watch out for anything based on your family medical history.

- You can find care within your insurance by asking your family.

- You can google family planning clinics – these clinics are used to seeing teens, often have low or no-cost options, and have experience with female issues.

- You can find a telehealth provider.

- Some urgent care centers will provide testing for STIs and emergency contraception pills.

Interactive Parts:

- If you could be anything, what would you be?

- What are your most important qualities for a friend?

- What is on your bucket list?

CHAPTER 4

~ ❖ ~

Maintenance

HEALTHY RELATIONSHIPS START WITH HEALTHY BOUNDARIES

Keeping the Vagina Clean/Healthy

- The vagina is pretty much self-cleaning, and some normal organisms live there that maintain the environment.

- When you wipe after peeing or pooping – it's important to start in the front, by your pubic hair, and wipe front to back towards the butt – this prevents bad things like bacteria from poop from getting to the front and causing problems or infection.

- There is no need for douching or any type of internal cleaning in the vagina, except for gentle soap and water during a shower – to the vulva – outside of the vagina.

- Media has made us think that sprays, gels, lotions, and deodorant are needed– they are NOT, and can be harmful – they can be very irritating to the skin on the outside and cause rashes and itching – NOT GOOD.

- The environment of the vaginal area is delicately balanced by the body to keep the pH level and good bacteria healthy and safe; when we add things like washes and douching, it changes that balance.

- If you think you have a very unusual or bad odor down there– see your doctor!

- It is never a good idea to use a type of food in the vagina – this sets the stage for infections and bad stuff (don't try yogurt inside the vagina for yeast infections).

Hair removal

- Hair was meant to be down there, there is no reason to remove it.

- Pubic hair has a purpose – it protects and cushions the vulva and vagina, keeping germs away.

- If you are going to remove hair – trim it first carefully with clean hair scissors.

Wax

- Waxing can be used for hair removal anywhere on the body, at home, or in the salon.

- Waxing can cause burns, inflammation, redness, burns, and infection if improperly done.

- Make sure if you wax your bikini area, you go to a licensed aesthetician, who does NOT double dip in the wax, makes you lay on a clean surface (preferably wax paper like the doctor's office), and uses gloves the whole time.

- Bikini wax – this removes hair from the areas not covered by a bikini.

- Brazilian Wax – this has become popular over the last 10 years, where all hair is removed from the private areas – bikini, vulva, near anus (butt), and in the front, on top of the pubic bone.

- Brazilian wax precautions – if this causes infection, inflammation, or burns – it can be very bad and painful because of the sensitivity of the area.

- Why would waxing cause an infection? There is a possibility of introducing new germs through double dipping or unclean practices to skin that may have cracks or openings. Also, infection can be acquired by burning the skin from too hot wax. Possible burns, double dipping, small cracks in the skin allowing bacteria in.

- Try to leave the skin alone for 24 hours – don't scrub it and also use over-the-counter pain reliever and cool compresses.

- If you think you have an infection or burn – GO see your healthcare provider.

Shave

- Prepare the skin – clean and exfoliate the skin and then use shaving cream if possible.

- Shave in the direction the hair grows.

- Always use a clean razor (don't share) and be mindful of bumpy soft skin that can be cut.

Lotions (depilatory)

- Examples of this are creams like Nair, which can be very irritating in the pubic area. These creams are not recommended because of the irritation they cause in sensitive areas.

Laser

- Find a licensed professional for this job.
- Perks – Permanent hair removal or reduction in the amount of hair.
- Disadvantages – can be painful, expensive, and can also cause irritation, burns, and inflammation.
- Sometimes it doesn't work with darker skin tones or lighter hair.

Questions

What do I use to clean my body in the shower?

Water and soap, preferably unscented.

Do I need to clean the inside of my vagina?
No.

If I am not sexually active, do I need to see a doctor? Will I have to get a pelvic exam?

It is a good idea and you will not be forced to do a pelvic exam.

Before you become sexually active is the BEST time to get the right information.

Look at the best options for you, review your family and medical history, and plan ahead.

What if I have bad pains, fatigue, headaches, or heavy bleeding with periods?

Go to see a healthcare provider for an evaluation.

What if I feel lumps in my breasts?

Go to see a healthcare provider for an evaluation.

Interactive Parts:

- How would you like people to describe you?

- What is your favorite quote and why?

- Where is your favorite place to be alone and think?

CHAPTER 5

~ ❖ ~

Infections

> "YOU WILL ALWAYS PASS FAILURE
> ON YOUR WAY TO SUCCESS."
> – **MICKEY ROONEY**

*F*irst, let's clarify that not ALL vaginal infections are sexually transmitted infections (STIs).

Many girls and women who have NEVER been sexually active can have certain types of infections.

These kinds of infections are yeast and bacterial infections.

Also, urinary tract infections can occur in any age female.

Any lumps or bumps should be looked at by a healthcare provider – we can get bumps from swollen glands, shaving, and cysts – just to name a few bumps that are NOT sexually transmitted.

However, all bumps, blisters, skin infections, or unusual things should be seen in person by a healthcare provider.

ALL unusual vaginal discharge or urinary pain or blood should be checked by a healthcare provider in-person at the clinic.

Why?

- We can test it in a lab
- We can look under a microscope, and test the pH
- We can make sure it is nothing else
- Based on our findings, we can treat it appropriately

> **Pro-tip:** These symptoms mentioned above can be caused by a variety of microorganisms. DO NOT treat every vaginal discharge with over-the-counter medication.

These infections deserve attention as they cause pain, discharge, and cramps, plus we can TREAT them.

Now, if you ARE sexually active, it is very important to be seen.

WORST CASE SCENARIO – you have a pelvic infection that leads to infertility.

Better case – you get diagnosed and treated and are fine.

Things to know

- Discharge that is not the usual color, texture, or scent – get it checked.

- Painful new cramps, abdominal pain – get it checked.

- Any new bumps, blisters, sores, ulcers, itching, redness, or external pain in the vaginal, on labia, or rectum – get it checked.

- Painful or bloody urination – get it checked.

The facts about STIs (focus on female symptoms and treatments)

Sexual activities – means anything where the genitals (a penis/anal area or vagina/anal area) touch the skin, mouth, or vagina and swap body fluids.

STI	Transmission	Prevention	Symptoms	Complications	Treatment
Gonorrhea	Through sexual activities	Using condoms	No symptoms or vaginal discharge/odor/irritation	Infertility and pelvic inflammatory disease	Treated with antibiotics
Chlamydia	Through sexual activities	Using condoms	No symptoms of vaginal discharge/odor/irritation, pain with urination	Infertility and pelvic inflammatory disease	Treated with antibiotics
Syphilis	Through sexual activities	Using condoms	No symptoms or sores in mouth or genitals	Fever, rash, and swollen glands. Can cause death if untreated	Treated with antibiotics
Herpes	Through sexual activities	Using condoms - helps decrease the chances of spreading	No symptoms, or red or painful or itchy blisters on labia, vagina or rectum	Can reoccur and can be spread to newborns during childbirth if untreated	Treated with antiviral pills, but these only decrease symptoms; it is not curable

HPV	Through sexual activities	Can be prevented with vaccination and condoms help decrease the chances of spreading	Flesh-colored bumps or warts – that can be painful or itchy blisters on labia, vagina, or rectum	Can reoccur	Treated with freezing, creams, lasers; it is not curable
Trichomoniasis	Through sexual activities	Using condoms	Smelly, green/yellow discharge	Pelvic inflammatory disease	Treated with antibiotics
HIV	Through sexual activities	Using condoms	Swollen lymph nodes, fevers, rash, oral infections	Can cause immune infections all over the body/AIDS and death if untreated	Treated with antiviral medicine to manage for life; it is not curable
Pubic Lice*	Through sexual activities	Abstinence from sexual activities	Itchy labia, vagina, or rectum	Discolored skin, secondary infections	Treated with pills

* These are bugs that are transferred from pubic hair and live and feed on the hair shaft.

A few words about Hepatitis B & C. Hepatitis is a liver disease spread through blood, bodily fluids, and needles (drug use). It can initially have mild or no symptoms and become a chronic infection. It's a virus, meaning it stays in the body forever, but there is a vaccination to prevent Hepatitis B.

If you are diagnosed with an STI and treated, you need to ABSTAIN from sexual activities.

Partners need to be treated at the SAME time while abstaining.

You can pass these infections back and forth if only one of you is being treated – sometimes partners lie or forget the medicine and you will not be cured if this happens.

New partners can lie about never having infections and give one to you.

After talking about all of these infections – hearing about the symptoms – the blisters, warts, the smelly discharge, the pain – the

possible consequences of not being able to get pregnant later on…..
and hearing some can't be prevented with condoms and you have
them for life – what does this mean???

It means every time you decide to have sexual activities with another
person – you put yourself at risk – you can imagine if that person has
had relations with many other people the risk goes up and up… but
many people don't tell the full story here – so you need to be extremely
picky, keep the number of people you have sexual activities with as low
as possible, and always use condoms to prevent many diseases.

Sexual Risk Calculator:

- There are calculators available on the web to estimate the number of
  people you are actually exposed to when having sex with people…

- When you have sexual relations with a person, you are exposed
  to every other person that they have had relations with also. So
  if you have had sex with one person = you are exposed to one
  person, if 2 people = exposed to 3 people, etc

  1= 1

  2=3

  3=7

  4=15

  5=31….

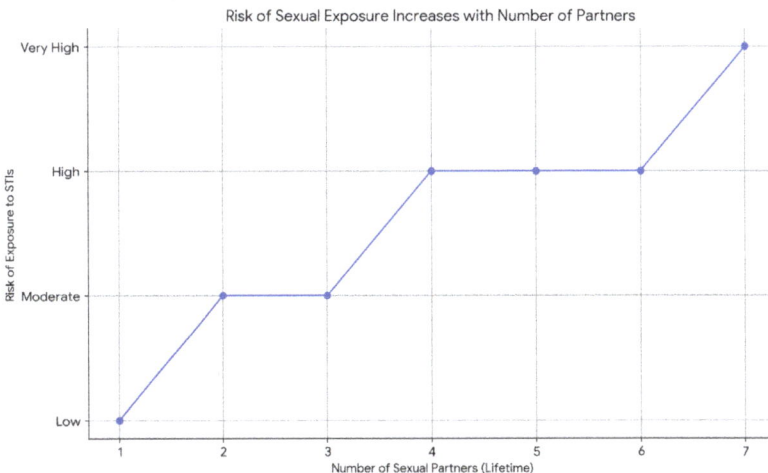

Risk of Sexual Exposure Increases with Number of Partners

Interactive Parts:

- Are you an early, on time or late person?

- What makes you feel really angry?

- What helps you calm down when you feel angry?

CHAPTER 6

~ ❖ ~

Preventing Pregnancy

"Even on your worst days, you are always worth love and respect. Don't ever settle for anything less."
-Hannah Irelan

What are the odds of getting pregnant?

- For women with periods, there is a chance of getting pregnant each month.

- If you are sexually active during the window of fertility, your chance greatly increases.

- If you are sexually active and not using birth control, you should be taking prenatal vitamins.

- **Important fact** – except for condoms, most of the birth control methods take time to work – so you can't expect to start the pill and be protected against pregnancy that day. Each method has different times to take effect and you NEED to make sure you know what those times are before you depend on it for pregnan-cy prevention.

- There are different types of birth control methods – those with and without hormones.

- Some women, because of certain medical issues or risk factors, are not allowed to take birth control with hormones. So, your medical provider will ask you about things like if you smoke, are over 35 years old, or have cancer, or heart issues/blood clots, or migraine.

- Make sure you honestly tell your provider about all your medical issues.

Methods of pregnancy prevention – good, bad, and awful ones...

- Withdrawal (pull out)

- Diaphragm

- Fertility Awareness Method (using calendar) - up to 27% chance of getting pregnant each year.

- Injection (shot)

- Birth control pills

- Patch

- Ring

- Implant (arm)
- Intra-uterine device (IUD)

We will review the most common methods for younger women.

1. Withdrawal (pulling out)

- This is a very tricky method of pregnancy prevention because it doesn't work well at all.
- It is based on the idea the male will pull out of the vagina right as he is about to ejaculate, or at the moment before the height of sexual pleasure – which is not when most males have good self-control.

So what goes wrong?

- The male is unable to get the timing right and sperm enters the vagina.
- There is pre-ejaculate (fluid with sperm that is released before ejaculation (orgasm)).
- The male can pull out but sperm are released all around the vagina and can get in.
- This is a BAD pregnancy prevention method and still risks you getting STIs.

2. Condoms

- Condoms alone, are not good pregnancy prevention.
- A younger age typically means higher rates of fertility or chances of becoming pregnant.
- If you are sexually active, there are two things to prevent – pregnancy + STIs.
- How do you do that? Pretty easy = condoms + some form of pregnancy prevention (birth control method).

- Condoms are great for stopping the spread of STIs like HIV, gonorrhea, and chlamydia.

- Condoms decrease the risk of STIs like herpes and warts, but they live in areas outside of condoms often, so you can still get them, even while using condoms.

- Condoms are not super user-friendly and are OFTEN put on the wrong way – and then they don't work.

- Condoms are often an afterthought after significant sexual activity has happened – they won't work.

3. Pills

- These methods contain hormones that prevent the normal cycles with ovulation from happening every month.

- It is best to go see a medical provider before starting to make sure you don't have any reasons to avoid this type of contraception.

- The lowest-risk pill is the progestin-only pill sold now over-the-counter.

- This pill is great, but works best ONLY if taken at the SAME time every day, like setting an alarm on your phone and making sure it happens EVERY DAY.

Progestin-only

- Most birth control pills have two hormones – this one has one which makes it a little tricker.

- You NEED to take it at the SAME time every day for it to work.

- Works by thickening the cervical mucous so that sperm can't enter the uterus and stops ovulation – but not all the time

Combined Birth Control Pills

- These are a mix of hormones, usually a progestin and estrogen type that essentially put your ovaries to sleep, so you don't ovulate and don't get pregnant (IF YOU TAKE THEM RIGHT).

- These pills need to be taken at the same time every day.

- Some of these pills have a few days where you bleed and some don't.

- AND it's okay if you don't bleed – that does not hurt you in any way.

- Use condoms to decrease the chances of pregnancy AND protect you against STIs.

- Some people can't take these because they are not safe with certain medical conditions – like blood clots – so you need to discuss this option with your provider.

- Some people experience headaches, bleeding in between periods, or breast tenderness.

- Some people get very light or no periods, decreased cramping, and decreased PMS.

- You need a prescription for these pills.

- **Danger Signs when taking birth control pills – go to the Emergency Room immediately;**

- **A**bdominal/belly pain – severe (concern for pregnancy in fallopian tubes or liver tumor)

- **C**hest pain or shortness of breath – severe (concern for heart issues or blood clot in the lung)

- **H**eadache – severe or weakness on one side (concern for blood clot or stroke)

- **E**ye issues – vision loss (concern for stroke or blood clot)

- **S**evere leg or calf pain (concern for a blood clot)

What if I travel?

- You can take birth control pills on a plane – keep the pack with the label of prescribing information.

- If you are changing time zones, there are no hard and fast rules – but you want to be as consistent as possible – you can always call your doctor for advice.

> **Pro tip** – pharmacists are all-knowing when it comes to medicines – for any questions, call your local pharmacist (or your healthcare provider) and ask anything about medication interactions, side effects, missing a dose, or forgetting pills a few days.

What if you forget a few days?

- Anytime you forget your pills for a few days, you are at risk of becoming pregnant and experiencing cycle irregularities like spotting, or an early period.

- If you are using your pills to prevent pregnancy, it is VERY important that you use a backup method – meaning – assume your pills aren't going to protect you and use a condom.

> **Pro tip**– many medications can interact with birth control pills also – prescribed or even over-the-counter supplements. It is important for you to ask your healthcare provider or pharmacist if medicines interact with birth control. You can also look up medication interactions on the web.

1. Patch (Twirla or Xulane)

- The patch is a small sticker with hormones put onto the skin (belly, back).

- It prevents pregnancy >90%.

- You change the patch every week.

- Like the pill, you can use the patch to skip a period.

- Still need a condom – DOESN'T protect against STIs.

- Some people have lighter or no periods and less cramps.
- Some people get headaches, sore breasts, or nausea.

2. Ring (Annovera, NuvaRing)

- The ring is a small flexible ring that a woman puts into the vagina for 3–6 weeks.
- It is effective >90%.
- You can use it to skip periods if you want.
- Some people experience headaches, nausea, lighter periods, less cramps.

3. Birth Control Shot (DepoProvera Injection)

- A shot is given by a medical provider every 12 weeks.
- It is effective >90%.
- Some people experience lighter, irregular, or no periods or nausea, headaches, weight gain, and sore breasts.
- People who take this are at a higher risk for bone loss.

4. Implants

- This is placed in the upper arm by a medical provider.
- Implants contain hormones so you may have irregular periods or none at all.
- It lasts for 5 years.
- Prevents pregnancy up to 99%.
- Use with Condoms = Pregnancy + STD prevention.

5. IUD

- This offers the most protection against pregnancy.
- These are tiny T–shaped devices with a string that are placed inside the uterus in a doctor's office.

- Some have hormones and some do not.

- They can last for 3–10 years, depending on the type of IUD.

- Prevent pregnancy up to 99%.

- You can get it removed anytime if you want to get pregnant.

- Some can make periods lighter, or even go away (IUD with hormones) and some can make them heavier (Copper IUD).

- The IUDs are a great option because there is once it is placed, you don't have to remember to take a pill or do anything every day. They are great for people who don't want to think about birth control frequently – this is one and done for years (just need to keep up with condom use).

- There is a tiny string (feels like a thread) that you can feel inside the vagina.

- They are uncomfortable to insert, but mostly the cramps go away with medicines like ibuprofen or acetaminophen.

- Condoms + IUD = pregnancy and STD prevention.

- No one has to know you have it.

- When it is time to replace it, it is removed in the office (usually takes a few minutes only) and a new one is placed.

- The BAD side – they DON'T protect against STDs – you still need to use a condom.

IUD picture

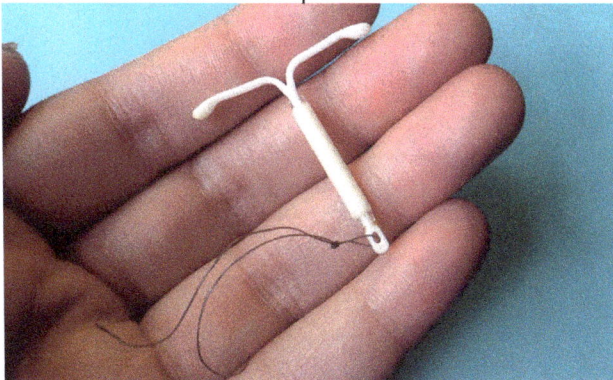

Saramirk, 2016

Uterus with Copper IUD Inside

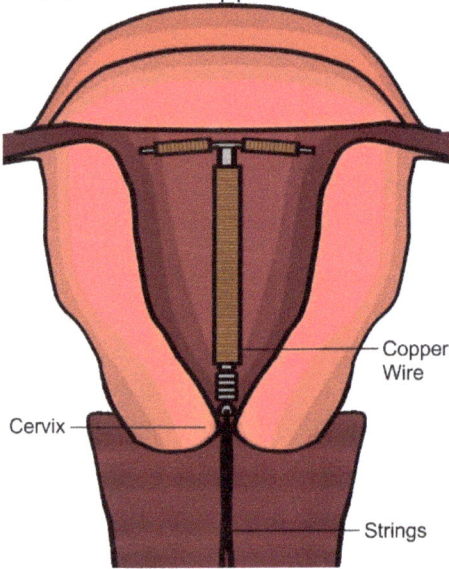

Copper
Wire

Cervix

Strings

Shipatadistance,2008

Copper IUD (Paraguard)

- Paraguard is an IUD without any hormones.

- It lasts 10 years as contraception.

- It uses a tiny piece of copper wrapped around it. As sperms hate copper, it makes the uterus very unfriendly to the sperm.

- Your periods may change – spotting, irregular, or heavier periods can happen.

Hormonal IUDs

- There are lots of kinds here that all work the same way – they thicken the mucous at the bottom of the uterus so sperm can't get in, and they can prevent the egg from leaving the ovary, so the sperm can't get to it.

- Because these IUDs have hormones – your periods can change– most people have spotting, light or no periods, and fewer cramps.

- These IUDs last anywhere from 3 – 8 years depending on the type.

- Listed are the brand names:
  - Skyla – 3 years
  - Kyleena – 5 years
  - Mirena or Liletta – 8 years

6. Emergency Contraception, Morning After Pill

- The EC is made for accidents– the condom broke, the condom wasn't used, the pill or other method was forgotten.
- There are a few kinds of EC – ulipristal acetate(Ella), levonorgestrel (Plan B), and many others or IUDs.
- The sooner you take it after sex, the better it works.
- If taken right, they can prevent pregnancy up to 80%.
- It works by delaying ovulation.
- It may delay your period, or make it heavier, lighter, or cause spotting.
- Take a pregnancy test if your period doesn't come within 2–3 weeks.
- These pills can interact with other medicines, so please ask your doctor or pharmacist if you are taking other medicines.
- Some clinics or family planning centers offer these at low to no cost, and most are covered by insurance.
- If you find yourself needing EC more than once, you should talk to your provider about better methods of birth control.

Levonorgestrel (Plan B)

- This has a few names, but it's a hormonal pill.
- It is sold over-the-counter at pharmacies without a prescription at any age.
- It needs to be taken within 3 days (72 hours) of unprotected sex.
- Works best if you weigh less than 165 lbs.

- Side effects can be headache and nausea.

- You can't take it within 5 days of taking another dose of EC.

Ulipristal acetate (Ella)

- This emergency contraception is used within 5 days (120 hours) of unprotected sex.

- These are sold by prescription, so you need to go to a doctor's office or clinic, or go online for a visit to get them.

- These hormonal pills work best if you weigh between 165–195 lbs.

IUD as an emergency contraceptive

- An IUD can be used as emergency contraception in some people.

- It is a device put through the vagina into the uterus to prevent pregnancy within 5 days of unprotected sex.

- Once the IUD is in, it will protect you against pregnancy for 8–10 years depending on which kind of IUD is used.

- Once placed, an IUD can prevent pregnancy up to 99%.

- You need to see your healthcare provider to see if this method is right and for it to be inserted.

Hormones and Pregnancy Later on

The idea with any hormone-type birth control is that it is reversible – meaning once you stop taking it, you should return to your normal cycles (assuming they were normal before the birth control) and your ability to get pregnant goes back to your normal ability.

It often takes a few months to return to your old cycle patterns.

Interactive Parts:

- What is one thing you will do differently than your parents?

- What would a perfect date look like to you?

- If you won $50,000, what would you do with it?

CHAPTER 7

~ ❖ ~

Consent

"LOVE YOURSELF. FORGIVE yourself. BE TRUE TO YOURSELF. BECAUSE HOW YOU TREAT YOURSELF SETS THE STANDARD FOR HOW OTHERS TREAT YOU."
– **STEVE MARABOLI**

- Consent can be a confusing word because many people think it means consent (saying yes) for sexual activities.

- Consent is actually saying yes, confidently to any activity that has the potential to make a person uncomfortable, like hugging, hand-holding, or kissing.

- Consent means there is a spoken agreement that both people involved want something to occur.

- Asking and receiving consent makes sure that each person feels safe, comfortable, and respected – which is the goal of a healthy relationship.

- If consent is NOT asked for and given, sexual activity can be considered an assault or rape. It is VERY important that both people clearly consent, and are willing to move forward.

Who asks for consent?

- Both people in a relationship should ask for consent when they want to do something to the other person – that can be a touch, a kiss, hand holding, or a hug.

- Consent needs to be asked every time this occurs – just because you have hugged or kissed this person before– does NOT mean it is okay to do it again without asking first.

- Because you are asking to do something with someone else's body – you need to be respectful that they may or may not feel comfortable doing things again.

People who CAN'T consent

- Underage (the legal age for consent for sex is different in every state).

- If a person doesn't fully understand what they are saying yes to.

- Sleeping people or those who passed out.

- People who have been drinking alcohol or doing drugs/other substances.
- People who are being coerced or forced, pressured, threatened, or bribed to consent – an example is if a person says to another person– "if you do this I won't share what you told me on social media", or "If you do this I will make you popular" or " if you don't do this, I will tell everyone you we had sex".

When to ask for consent?

- BEFORE you do whatever touching or action are you thinking.
- You must ask for consent and receive consent.

How do you ask for consent?

- Is this ok?
- Can I do…?
- Are you ok if I…?
- Would you like me to…?
- Can we…?
- Do you want to stop…?

How to say Yes to consent?

- It needs to be verbally spoken.
- It should be very clear.
- Say **Yes.**
- The person should seem enthusiastic and confident.

How to say NO to consent?

- Say NO.
- Shrug your shoulders.
- Be silent.
- Say Um.
- Say I am not sure.
- Say I don't know.
- Say I am not ready.
- Say not today.

Consent should be verbal to be clear – if you are asking for consent and the other person nods their head and you are unclear – ask for verbal consent to be very clear.

Consent is NOT granted by the body's natural response – meaning if you are close to a man and asking for consent and he has an erection – that is NOT consent, and the same for women – if a woman's nipple sticks out, that is NOT consent.

Clothing has NOTHING to do with consent – if a person is in a bathing suit or has on clothing that exposes their body – that is NOT consent.

When a person says "NO" to consent, the other person needs to be respectful – STOP and make sure the person saying NO knows that it is ok.

Consent can be taken back. If a person says "yes" but then feels uncomfortable and says "no", "let's stop" or something that signals they want to stop – YOU STOP. This is part of being a respectful partner.

When to step in…

- Reassure your friends that it is ok to do what only feels comfortable and they will be supported by you.

- If you see someone being pressured, or someone who is under the influence of drugs or alcohol – or any other nonconsensual situation – STEP IN and help.

- Watch out for friends being alone or in uncomfortable or unsafe situations.

CHAPTER 8

~ ❖ ~

The Gross Stuff

> "IF YOU ARE ALWAYS TRYING TO BE NORMAL, YOU'LL NEVER KNOW HOW AMAZING YOU CAN BE."
> **–MAYA ANGELOU**

Pee

- Urine should be light yellow, or clear if you are drinking enough water.

- It should not hurt to pee.

- If you have problems holding in your pee, burning while peeing, red or brown pee, or anything else that seems weird – please see your healthcare provider right away.

- Women can get urinary tract infections at any time in their lives, even if they do not have sex.

Poop

- People poop to get rid of waste in the body.

- How often people poop depends on many things – diet, exercise, hydration, illness.

- Most people poop once a day or more than once.

- What stool looks like can tell you about your health.

- Pooping should not be painful or bloody – if it is – see your healthcare provider ASAP.

- Constipation is when poop is hard like little rocks, and you have to push hard to get it out.

- Diarrhea is when poop is loose or watery and it comes out very easily.

- Normal poop should be in between constipation and diarrhea – soft, pretty easy to come out.

- Normal poop should be some shade of brown – not white, red, or black.

How to Keep Your Bowel Healthy

- Drink water every day – at least 60 oz.

- Manage stress – the brain and the bowels are deeply connected – and stress, depression, and anxiety can often cause problems with the bowels. If this is a problem for you, talk to your health-care provider.

- Eat fruits and vegetables.

- Eat fiber (vegetables and whole grains).

- Pre and Probiotics – good ways to get these are vegetables and a colorful diet – and foods like kombucha, kimchi, kefir, tempeh, and any fermented food like sauerkraut, greek yogurt, miso, sourdough bread. Yes, you can take a pill – but food is always better.

- Cleaning your colon – there is no need for enemas unless recommended by your doctor.

- There is no need to use baby wipes or any other special wipes instead of soft toilet paper.

- Always clean well – even small amounts of poop left behind can be irritating.

- Water Intake – At least 60 oz per day, but more if you are exercising or it is hot outside.

BRISTOL STOOL CHART

	Type	Description	Condition
	Type 1	Separate hard lumps	Very constipated
	Type 2	Lumpy and sausage like	Slightly constipated
	Type 3	A sausage shape with cracks in the surface	Normal
	Type 4	Like a smooth, soft sausage or snake	Normal
	Type 5	Soft blobs with clear-cut edges	Lacking fibre
	Type 6	Mushy consistency with ragged edges	Inflammation
	Type 7	Liquid consistency with no solid pieces	Inflammation

- Cabot Health, unknown date

Interactive Parts:

- What do your values look like?

- If you could spend an hour with one person, alive or dead, who would it be and why?

CHAPTER 9

~ ❖ ~

Eating Well

YOU MUST NEVER BE FEARFUL ABOUT WHAT YOU ARE DOING WHEN IT'S RIGHT.
— **ROSA PARKS**

Caffeine Intake

How much caffeine should I have?

- No amount of caffeine is needed.

- The highest amount of caffeine should be 100 mg per day.

  Example- Starbucks Pike's Place Roast 16 oz= 310 mg, Honest T tea= 86 mg, Coca-Cola= 34 mg, Celsius =200 mg, Starbucks Refresher = 50 mg

What are the bad effects of caffeine?

- Caffeine can give people a burst of energy but then can make you feel some pretty bad things – insomnia, nausea, increased heart rate, headache, restlessness, increased blood pressure, increased peeing, and many other effects.

- You can't taste or smell it, so it is hard to know when and how much you are having.

- Caffeine can make some mental conditions like anxiety and some physical conditions like heart issues, much worse.

- Caffeine is addictive and we have withdrawal symptoms when we stop like – anxiety, irritability, and being tired.

What drinks/foods have caffeine?

- Tea, coffee (even decaf has some caffeine), soda, hot chocolate, sports drinks, some lemonades, iced teas, chocolate coffee beans, chocolate, cocoa, some gums, some ice creams (coffee ice cream), tiramisu dessert

- Some vapes also contain caffeine

Food and Eating

- Unfortunately, our society has an unhealthy obsession with women's bodies and shapes.

- Whether it is trying to be the thinnest, most athletic, most tan, most muscular, most curvy, roundest bottom, perfect boobs, flat belly, or longest hair – we have all been exposed to the magazine article, Instagram, Snapchat pictures, and words of what you "should" look like per social media.

- The hard truth is our bodies are all different and not meant to look the same.

- Our goals need to first be body health. Lots of girls start dieting at way too early ages, pre-puberty – 8 and 9 years old.

So let's talk about diet – this word has a dirty sound – but a diet is a combination of the foods you eat every day.

What is a healthy diet or combination of foods????

- Foods that come from the Earth – fruits, vegetables
- Foods that only have a few ingredients
- Non-processed foods

What does healthy eating look like for a younger girl?

- The amount of food is going to increase based on the activity you do.

- More activity = more food

- What happens if you decrease food and increase activity? Weight loss.

- Where do we start? Find out if your weight and measurements are on target for your height and age.

  - If you are on target – make sure you are eating healthy foods most of the time.

  - If you are less than your target – you should try to add in healthy foods.

  - If you are past your target – try to think of foods that may be unhealthy to take out – but do it over time and increase activity.

- Nutritionists are people trained in foods/eating and can help you figure out if you need to change your diet to get to a healthier one.

- We all like to eat delicious food all the time.

- We should aim to eat healthy foods (non-processed foods) 80% of the time; 20% of the time, we can eat whatever we would like in normal quantities (the 80/20 rule).

- This rule permits us to eat any kind of food while maintaining a mostly healthy diet.

Best Combo

- Protein, fat, and carbohydrate at every meal and snack

- Eat three meals and a snack throughout the day.

- Intermittent fasting is not a good idea for growing women unless you are doing a 10–12 hour fast at night (meaning you are eating breakfast at 7 am and dinner by 7 pm, but still eat throughout the day).

Breakfast Food Ideas

- Eggs – scrambled, poached, fried, hard-boiled, omelets

- Breakfast meats – chicken sausage, turkey bacon

- Bread – whole grain or sourdough bread, protein pancakes/waffles

- Dairy – cottage cheese, yogurt (add fruits/nuts/seeds)

- Shakes – add fruits, nut butter, and veggies, to a base like milk (love Fairlife vanilla or chocolate milk with protein).

- Breakfast sandwiches – mix above

- Overnight oats with nuts/nut butter/seeds (need protein source)

Daily examples of healthy meals– lunch and dinners

- Avocado toast – sourdough bread with a teaspoon of olive oil, ¼ or ½ of avocado on top with an egg
- Overnight oats with yogurt, chia seeds, blueberries, cinnamon, and oats
- Sandwich – two scrambled eggs, turkey bacon, American cheese on wheat bread.
- Shake – Protein vanilla 1 cup, 1 cup spinach, 2 tablespoons almond butter and ½ banana
- Stir fry – a great way to add in meat (chicken/pork/steak) with a yummy sauce, and veggies of any kind – and put on top of brown rice, quinoa, and faro.
- **Proteins:**
- Fish – baked, grilled, or air fried – any kind with everything bagel seasoning, lemon, salt and pepper, and any kind of sauce
- Chicken, pork, or steak – baked, grilled, or air fried or sauteed
- Add in veggies and starch – any mix of veggies and starch ideas – potato, brown rice, wild rice, quinoa, farro, barley, buckwheat noodles
- For pasta – try to find one with added protein.

Meal substitutes/on-the-go

- Shakes and bars with protein are usually easy – watch out for added fake sugars (erythritol, stevia, aspartame).
- Usually works to bring food that does not need to be cold – jerky, peanut butter and jelly, granola bars, trail mix.

Snacks

Try to pair a protein, carbohydrate, and fat here too:

- Hummus/pretzels
- Cheese sticks and crackers

- Trail mix
- Peanut butter and celery/apple
- Yogurt/granola
- Nuts
- Smoothie
- Granola bar with protein
- Guacamole and carrots
- Roasted chickpeas
- Edamame

Interactive Parts:

- What is your favorite book and why?
- What is the best place your ever visited?

CHAPTER 10

~ ❖ ~

Sleeping Well

You attract what you are, not what you want. If you want great, then be great.

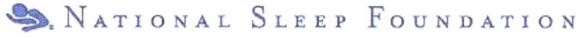

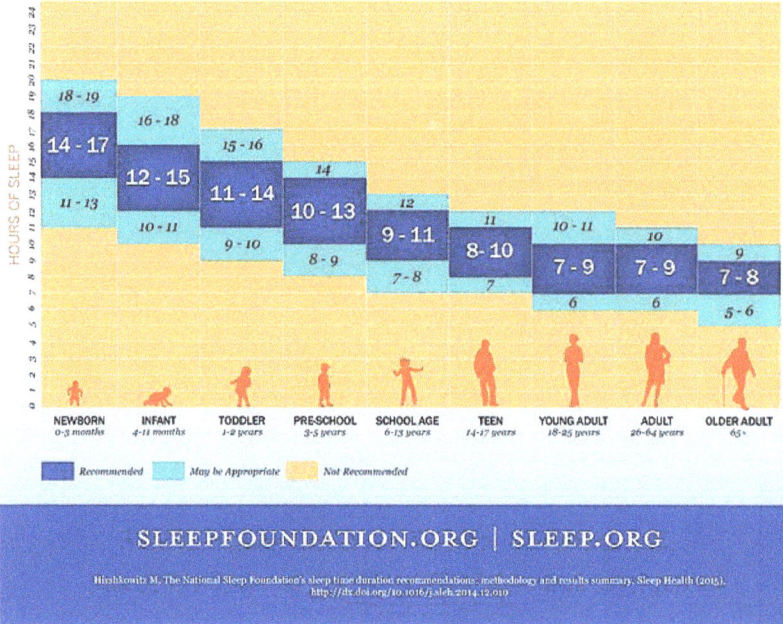

Sleep NSF, 2019

Sleep

What happens during sleep?

- Although you are resting – the brain is hard at work processing all the information from the day and creating memories for you.

- The heart, immune, and, metabolic system, and hormones are also working hard to keep your body in its best shape to grow, be healthy, and fight infection.

What is normal sleep?

- 8-10 hours per night

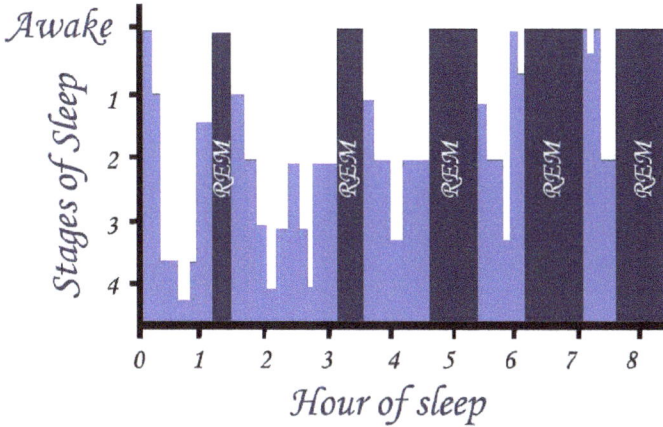

Bedzine, 2007

Stages of Sleep

Stage 1 – N1:

- The stage where you first fall asleep.
- Only lasts a few minutes

Stage 2 – N2:

- The next stage is where your body – muscles and brain – relax.
- You can be woken up easily.
- This stage lasts <30 minutes.

Stage 3 – N3

- Deep Sleep, N3, is when it is hard to wake up, and your brain and body slow down.
- Even though your brain has slowed, it is doing hard work to help your memories form and boost your creativity.

- Your immune system and hormones are also working hard during this stage to keep you healthy and keep normal growth and development on track.

- People spend about 1 hour in deep sleep throughout the night.

Stage 4 – Rapid Eye Movement (REM) Sleep

- The REM stage is the most important stage for a healthy brain, where memories, your daily experiences, and learning from the day come together.

- It is also the stage with the most dreams.

- People who get enough sleep, get about ¼ of their sleep or 2 hours or so in REM sleep.

What happens if you don't sleep?

- The front part of the brain is heavily affected by not sleeping and this is where we control impulses.

- So what does that mean? During the teenage years, this front area is forming memory, mood behavior, etc.

- Risky behaviors, and poor decision-making (people may choose to NOT wear seat belts, bike helmets, or condoms, they may drive drunk or use drugs, or make poor decisions with their bodies) if they don't have enough sleep.

- Also, medical issues like higher risk for cancer and heart disease may arise.

- Going without sleep for 17–24 hours (all-nighter) gives you a mental capacity and awareness that is equal to being drunk.

Sleep Issues

- There are some medical reasons why some people can't sleep.
- If you find yourself going without good sleep for a bit, please go see your healthcare provider and get checked.

How can I sleep better?

Sleep works best when you have a consistent pattern of going to bed and getting up around the same time every day.

Sleep Hygiene

DO – quiet dark room, same schedule every day, only sleep in your bed (don't do scrolling or homework), get exercise, get sunlight in the morning, eat at least 2 hours before bed

DON'T – have caffeine in the afternoon, nap, smoke

If you are lying in bed for more than 20 minutes, it is time to get up and try something different for a half hour – stretch, read a book, pray, meditate (don't get on your phone).

Can you make up for lost sleep?

- No – although it feels good to take a nap or sleep in on weekends – it doesn't allow for the same processes to happen in your body as if you sleep well every night.

What if I have to study all night for an exam?

You are better off sleeping and getting up early to study.

Does alcohol make you sleep better?

- No, actually you sleep worse after drinking alcohol.

Exercise

- Improves physical and mental health
- There are many kinds – aerobic and anaerobic
- Helps in maintaining a healthy weight
- Releases endorphins which decrease disease risk, anxiety, depression, and stress
- Increases energy, attention span, memory, sleep, endurance, and self–confidence

Interactive Parts:

- Which season is your favorite?

- If you had no plans for the summer and could do anything, what would you do?

CHAPTER 11

~ ❖ ~

Mental Health Issues

"MAY YOUR CHOICES REFLECT
YOUR HOPES, NOT YOUR FEARS."
– **NELSON MANDELA**

Managing Stress

- Stress will be in your life forever in many forms – friendships, work, school – the sooner you can learn to manage stress, the better off you will handle it for the rest of your life.

- If stress feels so overwhelming that you can't figure out how to handle it, or it isn't allowing you to do your normal stuff – concentrate, sleep, relax – please see a mental health counselor/therapist. They can assess what's going on and give you lots of tools and ways to help with stress.

- Social media/scrolling/watching TikTok will BRING ON stress, so please don't use it to relieve stress.

- Find your happy place

  - Being in nature – walking on the beach or outside. When we are in nature, stress decreases, we feel increased happiness and well–being, better energy, and have clearer thinking.

  - Find a hobby – audiobooks, dancing, painting, running, coloring, collecting something

  - Use mental breaks – yoga, meditation, prayer

  - Volunteer – brings focus from yourself to others.

  - Watch movies

  - Make a vision board, write goals, and keep it positive.

Younger women can have a mix of emotions and moods that change every day – how do we know what is normal and what is not normal for us and for our friends?

Physical clues to emotional problems

- Feeling tired all the time
- Sleeping too much or too little
- Changes in eating or appetite (can be gaining or losing weight)
- Noticing self–inflicted physical injuries
- Using drugs or alcohol

- Slower thinking or speaking
- Lots of physical problems (headaches, pain)

Behavioral clues to problems

- Noticing frequent anger, anxiety, or sadness
- Decreasing social activities
- Feeling hopeless or crying frequently
- Isolating from friends and family

If you or your friends have these signs, it is VERY important to seek help right away from a healthcare provider or counselor.

If you or any of your friends are thinking about hurting themselves– Call or text 988, which is the US Suicide and Crisis hotline available 24/7 (FREE and CONFIDENTIAL), or Crisis for Teens text the number – 4HELP (44375) and text the word "safe" and you can start a conversation

For anyone who is suicidal, call 911 and stay with the person until help arrives

Eating and Food Issues

- During teens and early twenties, we can start to see eating disorders come into play.

What are eating disorders?

- Any combination of restrictive eating, binging on food or vomiting, or laxative abuse are classified as eating disorders.
- Some people with eating disorders will be very underweight, while other people can be normal weight or overweight.
- Eating disorders have really bad effects on the body and can even lead to death.

Warning signs of an eating disorder

- Preoccupation with food, weight, appearance, eating
- Feeling anxiety/stress/guilt around eating – before, during, or after
- Weight changes – gaining or losing weight
- Very critical of self or putting down body or personality

If you have a friend, or you feel like you may have an eating disorder – it is important to get help right away.

- Eating Disorder Helpline
  - 1–888–375–7767
  - Mon– Fri
  - 9 am–9 pm

Interactive Parts:

- **What is your favorite childhood memory?**

RESOURCE LIST

1. Suicide & Crisis Line- Call, text or chat 988, 24/7 https://988life-line.org/chat/

2. Substance Abuse & Mental Health Services Call 1800-662-4357 24/7 https://988lifeline.org/chat/

3. Disaster Distress Helpline- for crisis after a disaster Call 1800-985-5990

4. Teen Help Line 800-852-8336 or text 839863. Evenings only 6-10 pm Pacific Time https://www.teenline.org/

5. National Alliance on Mental Illness 1 800-950-6462 Mon-Fri 10 am-10 pm

6. Human Trafficking Hotline 1 888-373-7888 Text 233733 24/7

7. National Domestic Violence Hotline 1 800-799-7233 or Text 88788 24/7

8. National Association for Anorexia and Associated Disorders 1 888-375-7767 9 am-9 pm Mon- Fri

9. Alcoholics Anonymous 1 888-425-2666 8 am-6 pm Mon-Fri

10. LGBTQ Talkline 1 800-246-7743

Websites

Periods, Birth Control, Wellness

Teen Talk

https://teentalk.ca/learn-about/birth-control-2/

Teen Health and Wellness

https://teenhealthandwellness.com/

Center for Young Women's Health

https://youngwomenshealth.org/

Amaze- videos explaining health, puberty, sex, etc.

https://amaze.org/us/

Planned Parenthood- Birth Control Page

https://www.plannedparenthood.org/learn/teens/stds-birth-control-pregnancy/what-do-i-need-know-about-birth-control

Web MD Birth Control Page

https://www.webmd.com/sex/birth-control/birth-control-teens

Healthy Children Birth Control Page

https://www.healthychildren.org/English/ages-stages/teen/dating-sex/Pages/Birth-Control-for-Sexually-Active-Teens.aspx

Girls Health- body, fitness, nutrition, bullying

https://www.girlshealth.gov/

Stop Smoking, Vaping

https://truthinitiative.org/thisisquitting

Apps

Food

- My fitness pal
- My Net Diary

Mood

- Headspace
- Calm
- Smiling mind
- Hmm- healthy minds

Period

- Flo
- Clue
- Spot on
- Luna

Medication Interaction Checker

Web MD

> https://www.webmd.com/interaction-checker/default.htm

Drugs.com

> https://www.drugs.com/drug_interactions.html

Interesting and Inspiring Ted Talks

Brene Brown- the Power of Vulnerability

Courtney Ferrell- The Secrets to an Extraordinary Life

Angela Duckworth- Grit: The Power of Passion and Perseverance

Simon Sinek- Start With Why

Julian Treasure-How to Speak So That People Want to Listen

Amy Cuddy-Your Body Language May Shape Who You Are

Cynthia Ong-Redefining How We Love

Kelly McGonigal-How to Make Stress Your Friend

Sharon Livingston- 8 Signs of a Toxic Friendship

REFERENCES:

ACOG (2022a) *Dysmenorrhea: Painful periods, ACOG*. Available at: https://www.acog.org/womens-health/faqs/dysmenorrhea-painful-periods (Accessed: 19 June 2024).

ACOG (2022b) *The menstrual cycle: Menstruation, ovulation, and how pregnancy occurs, ACOG*. Available at: https://www.acog.org/womens-health/infographics/the-menstrual-cycle (Accessed: 19 June 2024).

AHA (2022) *Most of the nation's teens aren't getting enough exercise, www.heart.org*. Available at: https://www.heart.org/en/news/2020/04/09/most-of-the-nations-teens-arent-getting-enough-exercise (Accessed: 19 June 2024).

AHA (2022) *Most of the nation's teens aren't getting enough exercise, www.heart.org*. Available at: https://www.heart.org/en/news/2020/04/09/most-of-the-nations-teens-arent-getting-enough-exercise (Accessed: 19 June 2024).

Baum, H. (2021) *The endocrine system*. Available at: https://www.palmbeachstate.edu/slc/Documents/AandPch16LecturePearson.pdf (Accessed: 20 June 2024).

Bedzine (2007). REM graph. https://www.flickr.com/photos/beds/445253350 Accessed 15 July 2024

Birth control pills rawpixelhttps://www.rawpixel.com/image/5920306

Breehl, L. (2023) *Physiology, puberty, StatPearls [Internet]*. Available at: https://www.ncbi.nlm.nih.gov/books/NBK534827/ (Accessed: 19 June 2024).

CDC (2022) *Youth physical activity guidelines, Centers for Disease Control and Prevention*. Available at: https://www.cdc.gov/healthyschools/physicalactivity/guidelines.htm (Accessed: 19 June 2024).

Cabot Health, unknown date. Bristol Stool Chart. https://commons.wikimedia.org/wiki/File:Bristol_stool_chart.svg Accessed 15 July 2024.

Ciell.(2007). Injection for Birth Control. https://commons.wikimedia. org/wiki/File:Prikpil.JPG, (Accessed 15 July 2024)

Cycle Syncing Nutrition and Exercise. (2023, April 3). Cleveland Clinic. https://health.clevelandclinic.org/nutrition-and-exercise-through-out-your-menstrual-cycle

Dorwart, L. (2023, May 23). *Everything You Need to Know About How to Eat and Exercise During Your Menstrual Cycle.* Health. https://www.health. com/cycle-syncing-7500732

Dr. Anita Dhanorkar, B. (2023) *What is the normal cycle for menstruation? 3 phases, period last, changing, MedicineNet.* Available at: https://www.med-icinenet.com/what_is_the_normal_cycle_for_menstruation/article. htm (Accessed: 19 June 2024).

Emmanuel, M. (2022, December 11). *Tanner stages.* StatPearls [Internet]. https://www.ncbi.nlm.nih.gov/books/NBK470280/

Hiller-Sturmhöfel S, Bartke A. The endocrine system: an overview. Alcohol Health Res World. 1998;22(3):153-64. PMID: 15706790; PMCID: PMC6761896.

Isometrik. (2008). Image. https://commons.wikimedia.org/wiki/ File:MenstrualCycle3.png

Miyamoto M, Shibuya K. Exploring the relationship between nutrition-al intake and menstrual cycle in elite female athletes. PeerJ. 2023 Sep 25;11:e16108. doi: 10.7717/peerj.16108. PMID: 37780394; PMCID: PMC10538277.

Nahas, D. (n.d.). *EATING DISORDER FACT SHEET FOR EDUCATORS.* Retrieved July 7, 2024, from https://smhp.psych.ucla. edu/pdfdocs/edfactsheet.pdf

OASH (2021) *Menstrual cycle, Menstrual Cycle | Office on Women's Health.* Available at: https://www.womenshealth.gov/menstrual-cycle (Accessed: 19 June 2024).

Parenthood, P. (n.d.). *Birth Control Methods & Options: Types of birth control.* Planned Parenthood. https://www.plannedparenthood.org/learn/ birth-control

Pereira HM, Larson RD, Bemben DA. Menstrual Cycle Effects on Exercise-Induced Fatigability. Front Physiol. 2020 Jun 26;11:517. doi: 10.3389/fphys.2020.00517. PMID: 32670076; PMCID: PMC7332750.

Reed, B.G. (2018) *The normal menstrual cycle and the control of ovulation, Endotext [Internet]*. Available at: https://www.ncbi.nlm.nih.gov/books/NBK279054/ (Accessed: 19 June 2024).

Saramirk.(2016). IUD. https://commons.wikimedia.org/wiki/File:Mirena_IUD_with_hand.jpgAccessed 15 July 2024

ShipataDistance(2002). A diagram showing a copper IUD placed in a uterus. https://commons.wikimedia.org/wiki/File:Iuddiagram.jpg Accessed 15 July 2024

Sleep NSF. (2019). Sleep. National Sleep Foundation. https://commons.wikimedia.org/wiki/File:NSF_Sleep_Duration_Recommendations_Chart.jpg Accessed 15 July 2024

Sleep Foundation (2023) *Teens and sleep, Sleep Foundation*. Available at: https://www.sleepfoundation.org/teens-and-sleep (Accessed: 19 June 2024).

Sleep Problems in Teens. (n.d.). UCLA Health. Retrieved June 19, 2024, from https://www.uclahealth.org/medical-services/sleep-disorders/patient-resources/patient-education/sleep-and-teens

Sung E, Han A, Hinrichs T, Vorgerd M, Manchado C, Platen P. Effects of follicular versus luteal phase-based strength training in young women. Springerplus. 2014 Nov 11;3:668. doi: 10.1186/2193-1801-3-668. PMID: 25485203; PMCID: PMC4236309.

Teens and sleep: Why you need it and how to get enough. Paediatr Child Health. 2008 Jan;13(1):69-72. doi: 10.1093/pch/13.1.69. PMID: 19119357; PMCID: PMC2528821.

Teixeira, J., Rueda, B.R., and Pru, J.K., Uterine Stem cells (September 30, 2008), StemBook, ed. The Stem Cell Research Community, StemBook, doi/10.3824/stembook.1.16.1, http://www.stembook.org.

Thensf. (2024, May 10). *What To Know About Teens and Sleep*. National Sleep Foundation. https://www.thensf.org/what-to-know-about-teens-and-sleep/

Thompson B, Almarjawi A, Sculley D, Janse de Jonge X. The Effect of the Menstrual Cycle and Oral Contraceptives on Acute Responses and Chronic Adaptations to Resistance Training: A Systematic Review of the Literature. Sports Med. 2020 Jan;50(1):171-185. doi: 10.1007/s40279-019-01219-1. PMID: 31677121.

Todd, N. and Black, A. (2020) *Contraception for adolescents, Journal of clinical research in pediatric endocrinology*. Available at: https://www.ncbi.nlm.nih.gov/pmc/articles/PMC7053440/ (Accessed: 19 June 2024).

UCSF (no date) *Normal menstrual cycle: UCSF Center for Reproductive Health, UCSF*. Available at: https://crh.ucsf.edu/about-fertility/normal-menstrual-cycle (Accessed: 19 June 2024).